How to Improve Your Vision Naturally

Strategies and Exercises to Restore Your Eyesight

Nick Stanton

Published by:
Nick Stanton and Random Technologies
4409 HOFFNER AVENUE, SUITE 347
Belle Isle, FL 32812
www.SparrowPublication.com

Disclaimer

This book is intended as reference material and not as a medical manual to replace the advice of your eye physician or to substitute for any treatment prescribed by your eye physician.

If you are ill or suspect that you have a medical problem, we strongly encourage you to consult your medical, health or other competent professional before adopting any of the suggestions in this book or drawing inferences from it. If you are taking prescription medication, you should never change your diet (for better or worse) without consulting your eye physician.

This book and the author's opinions are solely for informational and educational purposes.

Thank You for Choosing our Book!

Your purchase means a lot to us, and we hope this report on Improving Your Vision Naturally meets your expectations.

Table of Contents

Paving the Way So You Can See – Naturally!

Optometry is a booming business. Millions today have some form of corrective vision aid. Contacts, glasses and night time or reading glasses (also called "cheaters") -- these are all used to correct vision. These products help their users to see better but do not actually improve eyesight. In fact, eyewear often creates dependencies without addressing the users' ability to improve their vision.

A myth of irreversibility surrounds eyesight. People tend to think that once they need glasses, they'll always need glasses. But it's not true! There is much that can be done to restore your vision naturally if you've suffered eyesight damage. It's unfortunate that people never correct their vision because they depend on vision aids due to a misguided belief in this myth. However, you don't have to be one of these people.

This book details some of the best methods for improving your vision naturally – without surgery. From medication to regular dietary needs, there is much we can do on a daily basis that affects how we see. This book is chock full of facts that will surprise and even inspire you.

Review sections as necessary to remind yourself about the ways you can work to correct your vision naturally. As you read, try the tips! You will be amazed at the improvement you can make to your eyesight.

Introduction

Warning: The information in this guide is comprehensive but not intended to replace medical attention. If you are currently experiencing vision loss problems, seek a physician's help BEFORE treating yourself.

Eyesight is one of the most important and overlooked of our senses. People don't realize how their eyesight changes as they age. By the time they realize something is amiss, their sight has worsened dramatically.

Eyesight loss typically progresses step by step. First, images aren't as clear as they once were. Then, you find yourself stepping back to read a sign. Yet it's only after truly struggling with reading will most people make an appointment with their optometrist. Optometrists are skilled at finding solutions to help you see better immediately. Glasses and contacts relieve discomfort but few optometrists go further than prescribing eyewear. Often they do not tell what you can do to improve your vision naturally. Over-reliance on these aids can actually worsen your vision. Your eyes will not exert themselves since the optometrist's prescription does the work for you!

This book is intended to act as a guide to those who need corrective vision aids. We'll help you to exercise your eyes while you're seeking the advice of your optometrist.

Let's get started!

Straining Your Eyes – How Do YOU Do It?

Our eyes are one of the most abused organs in our body. We work them hard continually yet few of us actually take care of them properly. This book will look at how you can better maintain your eyesight. First, you need to see how you contribute to your eyesight issues.

Take a moment to think about how you usually spend your day. Are you busy all the time? Do you eat right? How stressed are you? The number one culprit of eyesight impairment is your health. While this may come as a surprise you'll see how these factors and more can contribute to eyesight problems.

Let's begin when you were a kid. Research suggests that children all start with a baseline of vision that then deteriorates as they age. What happens as children age? They develop habits and behavioral patterns that either help or hurt their vision. Many of these habits are created and adopted at school.

That's right -- school. How has the educational system helped or hurt your eyes? The mere fact that it's a system has implications. As a child you began learning long before you set foot into a classroom, such as how to walk, how to talk, where to go or not go by yourself. All these were learned at your own pace and when you were interested in learning them. So why is school different?

At school, children are forced into a new routine and subjected to social, academic and scheduling pressures. They're told what they will learn and when. When you were younger you had much more control over learning, if only on a need-to-know basis. However, at school you were required to memorize and regurgitate several specifically outlined subjects. You're even given a time frame to complete your education and punished if you don't maintain the learning pace of your peers! All these pressures accumulate, stressing both your body and your eyes.

At these especially vulnerable younger ages, children work hard to please the adults around them. This is true even when they strain themselves. One of the main organs visibly affected is the eyes. When tired, you should relieve your eyes but if you've missed an assignment deadline the chances of relaxing are slim and none. School age children learn that this strain is just a normal part of 'working hard' and so it becomes just another item in a long list of poor eyesight habits they adopt.

So what are some of the other primary lifestyle problems that lead to eyesight issues?

- Bad diet
- Alcohol abuse
- Boredom (which leads to other factors that influence eyesight like posture or strain)
- Inadequate or excessive lighting
- Extended screen exposure (TV, computer, iPhone)
- Forcing yourself to read when you are tired
- Poor posture
- Straining your eyes to see
- Stress

You might panic looking at the items on this list but everyone has at least a few poor lifestyle habits that lead to eyesight issues. What's the good news? You can change your routine! There isn't any one reason causing your eyesight issues. While improvement won't happen overnight, the suggestions found in this book will help you break habits that damage your sight.

Rest assured that changing these habits does help reverse at least some of the damage! If you're prepared to alter your lifestyle, given time you will see more clearly. Be patient and work at a pace that feels comfortable to you.

How and Why You Should Relax Your Eyes

We understand your eyes don't just relax themselves. This chapter examines how and why you should work regularly to relieve your eyes.

How to Relax Your Eyes

Find a calm, quiet place where you can feel at peace. Block some time out, seat yourself, close your eyes and focus on serene tranquility. Visualization techniques are helpful; picture a place that makes you feel restful and calm. Or just sit and allow yourself to recognize the inner peace within yourself. Take a minute to slow your breathing, focusing on deep quality breaths that promote relaxation.

Now that you're calm, focus on the darkened back of your eyelids. Stay in this position until you feel utterly relaxed. Be sure to set aside time to relax before resuming your normal activities.

When you finally return to your appointed rounds, you'll find that just by sitting down for a few minutes has sharpened your focus. This is one way you can improve your vision.

Why You Should Relax Your Eyes

Allowing your eyes to relax can be a very efficient use of your time. You may be stunned to learn how eye strain affects your body. If you start taking care of your eyes you will see improvement in not only your sight but reduce headaches and stress while improving your sense of overall well-being.

The science behind relaxation is simple. Relaxing reduces tiredness, improves vision and refocuses you for more work in the day. To maximize employee efficiency, many employers even set time aside so their employees can relax.

After you did the exercise above, you likely noticed that you were able to see considerably better after relaxing. The reason? You took time to remove stress and instead focus on relaxation. One significant benefit of relaxation: the more you practice, the less time it takes to relax.

Since not all of us have the time or space for a daily tranquil escape, here are some shorter exercises that should also help to improve your vision.

How to Relax Your Eyes In a Hurry

Eye Relaxation Exercise # 1 -- Take a minute to look away from the computer screen (read the instructions first). Notice something in the distance and focus on it. Next, find something else either further or closer away. Allow your eyes to completely focus on the objects. Permitting your eyes to refocus helps maximize your ability to concentrate.

Eye Relaxation Exercise # 2 -- Look away from the screen again but now just concentrate on blinking. Blinking helps the eyes lubricate, preventing strain.

Several more exercises are presented throughout this guide but these two help you realize why taking care of your eyes is so critical.

The Good, the Bad and the Shocking Truths about Vision Problems

There are many causes for your deteriorating vision. Stress, lifestyle, diet and even medication can affect eyesight. What medications are you taking? Do you know which ones impact your vision? How stressed you are? Are you aware how stress affects your health and vision? Do you know the connection between carrots and eyesight? How does your current diet contribute to the condition of your vision? This chapter examines some myths and realities about vision loss.

Vision Loss Myths

Before we look at these myths, I want to encourage you to take notes on how they may currently affect your vision. If you mistakenly believed an activity is good for your vision -- but isn't -- then you were wasting both time and effort in attempting to improve your eyesight.

Some of the most popular myths are:
- Contact lenses help nearsightedness
- Night lights hurt a toddler's vision
- Reading in the dark is bad for you
- Over the counter glasses are bad for your eyes
- Sitting too close while watching TV damages your eyesight
- Carrots will give you good eyesight

The last item on the list may surprise you but you should know the truth rather than believe a myth is reality. Myths are often based on tiny bits of truth and then promptly blown out of proportion. Consider the carrot myth. Carrots *are* good for you; they just don't improve your vision. This vegetable by no means should be excluded from your diet but it alone won't be responsible for improving your eyesight.

It's worth noting that none of the items on the list above hurt your eyesight. They just aren't as helpful as you may have thought. The bottom line is to recognize the myths as well as reality about vision loss.

True (and Surprising) Facts about Vision

- Reading in the dark CAN strain your eyes and should be done with caution
- Over the counter glasses can work for the people they were designed to help but this may not include you
- Contact lenses can create dependency on vision aids that discourages you from improving your vision naturally

So take the grains of truth and discard the myths. The best way to improve vision? Give your eyes time to relax. Don't let myths keep you from improving your vision. What's the best way not to be misled by these myths? Do your research! Study the particular problem affecting your eyesight and learn how to treat it. Or research facts to verify them and separate them from myths.

By eliminating myths and focusing on small exercises that help your vision you will be on your way to strengthening your eyesight naturally.

Eye Relaxation Exercise # 3 -- Close your eyes and let them relax until all you can see is the darkened back of your eyelids. Now open.

Even small relaxation techniques like the one above make a tremendous difference in the quality of your vision.

How Will I Know When My Vision Is Improving?

Just as vision disappears slowly and subtly, improvement progresses the same. However, you can measure how your vision is improving. When you shift focus, notice how long it takes. As you do more of these exercises, you may be able to hold focus longer or see easier from a distance. You may not have recognized vision improvement if you hadn't taken time to test.

Glasses, Contacts, Vision Aids: Do They Help or Hurt?

Those who wear glasses frequently find that sometimes their vision is better without glasses. Other times it only seems to function with them. As we have discussed already, glasses do not actually correct your eyesight. They act as a corrective aid that helps you to see without improving your sight.

So do glasses help or hurt?

The short answer is neither. They do help you to temporarily see but don't help correct your vision. They do hurt you by creating a dependence on corrective aids but don't actually cause damage to the eye. *It was never the goal of glasses to 'cure'!*

If you doubt this, pick a day where you can stay home and remove your glasses. (Remember to stay safe.) A few hours later, see how you feel and how well you see.

The next step is to complete the following exercise that will actually help you improve your vision.

Eye Relaxation Exercise #4 --Put your glasses back on for a few minutes and find an item with many words. This item can be a book or even a picture but ideally will have varying sizes of text.

Before continuing, take time to focus on relaxing by using the techniques above or others.

Once you're sufficiently relaxed, look at the line with varied sizes of words. Begin with the large words, then move to the smaller ones and try to read them. Then remove your glasses and try to read the line again. Focus on these words until your vision blurs. When your vision blurs, stop. This tells you the state of your vision without unnecessarily straining your eyes.

Eye Relaxation Exercise #5 -- Repeat the eye relaxation from earlier, this time *with variation*. Cover your eyes with your hands, keeping your lids closed. Do not put pressure on your eyes or you could cause further damage. Once again, you will be more relaxed the darker you let your eyes become.

Now, slowly remove your hands from your eyes and open them again. Try to read the same line of words from before again until the point of blurriness. This test will act as a gauge for you. If you can read more the second time, then you know it's possible to improve your vision with exercise and effort.

Keep in mind that when you start these exercises you will probably have limited improvement. But over time the goal is to gain more ability with your eyesight. In fact, as you work with these exercises, you will start to see long term improvement and hopefully need your glasses less.

The goal is not to be rid of your glasses! You will likely always need your glasses at times. You want to improve your vision as best you can.

Medications That Damage Your Eyes

Medications can be very beneficial. When you have lingering flu, you're grateful for antibiotics to treat your malady. So grateful in fact, you probably don't take time to consider what those drugs do to your body.

Many medications are fine and perfectly safe for your eyes. However, there are some commonly prescribed drugs that go unquestioned yet cause trouble for your eyesight. This chapter surveys some of the most harmful drugs and their effects on vision to help you make an informed decision about their use.

Drugs Linked to Cornea Damage

- Chloroquine
- Hydroxychoroquine
- Quinacrine

These drugs are all anti-malarial drugs but have also been linked to side effects such as glare sensitivity, light sensitivity, blurred halos around sources of light and more. However it's worth noting that these effects disappear with no permanent damage after ceasing use.

Drugs Linked to Retina Damage

- Blood pressure medication – Clonidine/Catapres
- Hydroxchloriuine sulfate (Plaquenil) – Popular arthritis treatment
- Non-Steroidal Anti-Inflammatory Drugs (NSAIDS) – all kinds. The best known NSAIDs are aspirin, ibuprofen and naproxen. Damage is linked to long term exposure of these drugs. However, don't panic about taking a single pill.
- Thioridazine

Drugs Linked To Blood Clots

- Androgen hormone replacements
- Estrogen

Drugs Linked To Hemorrhaging of the Eye

- Antibiotic - Amphotericin B
- Anti-coagulants – Anisidione, Coumadin, Hesparin
- Alzheimer's treatment - Cholesterase inhibitors
- Non-Steroidal Anti Inflammatory Drugs (NSAIDs)
- Painkillers
- Pentoxifylline (blood clots)
- Venlafaxine (anti-depressant)

Drugs Linked To Cataracts and Macular Degeneration

- Antidepressants
- Antibiotics – Fluroquinone, Terbinafine, Mefloquine
- Antihistamines
- Eretinate
- Glucocorticoids (Prednisone)
- Isoretinoin
- NSAIDS – Advil, aspirin, ibuprofen, meclofen
- Oral contraception (the pill)
- Steroids
- Sulfa drugs
- Tranquilizers

Drugs Linked To Glaucoma

- Antidepressants
- Fenfluramine
- Gastric antispasmodics
- Mirtazapine
- NSAIDS
- Simvastatin
- Steroids (Prednisone)
- Venlafaxine

Steroids

Steroids should be taken only as a last resort. Ask your physician about alternatives (perhaps hydrocortisone) before accepting a steroid prescription. If you are taking steroids, supplement your diet! You will need loads of extra vitamins, particularly beta-carotene, C and E.

Prevalence of These Medications

Most of us have used many of these substances (NSAIDS, for example) at one point or another. They do provide pain relief in many cases and they are often eagerly and gratefully accepted. This chapter is here so you can make an informed choice before taking these medications. Are the potential side effects worth it?

If you are wondering how often these effects occur, or the effects of your current medications, consult the documentation included with the drug's packaging or the pharmacist who dispensed them. The information is there but you will not find it by blithely taking pills while ignoring the facts surrounding these remedies.

Finally, there will be times when you simply cannot avoid these medications/substances. Just know the dangers and if possible how to counteract their effects to keep your vision at its highest efficacy. If knowledge is power, this information should give you confidence that you're taking charge of your healthy eyesight.

Conditions That Can Affect Your Eyesight

Remember: The information in this book is <u>NOT</u> a substitute for medical advice.

At any given moment there are several conditions that could affect a person's eyesight, some relatively benign and those that can cause severe damage. This chapter and the ones that follow survey several different conditions (although this is not a comprehensive list) and how you can best manage each of them to reverse damage or at least prevent further harm.

A final warning -- don't self-diagnose. Optometrists are licensed to tell you which of these conditions you may have. Consult them if you think you're suffering from one or more of these maladies.

The conditions covered are:
- Myopia
- Presbyopia
- Dyslexia
- Floating objects in the line of vision
- Glaucoma
- Macular degeneration

Myopia

Myopia aka short-sightedness is the condition wherein people see objects nearby very easily but struggle with those farther away. Myopic vision blurs items together at a distance rather than refocusing on them. This occurs when the eyeballs are elongated lengthwise (more oval than round). There are three different types of myopia:

Myopia from Shortly After Birth

This type of myopia describes children who develop the condition while still wearing diapers.

Cause? The current wisdom suggests that medications (particularly anti-hypertensive drugs), cataracts, or diabetes can lead to this type of myopia.

*Note: Despite this type of myopia appearing shortly after birth, myopia is not genetically linked from parent to child.

Myopia in a 5 - 10 Year Old Child

Causes? There are two subcategories of myopia present at this time in a child's life -- axial and refractive. Axial myopia is the situation described above, the elongation of the eyeball (oval, not round). In contrast, refractive myopia involves a difference in corneal strength, resulting in the distortion of vision at a distance.

Mercifully, this type of myopia is most common. Fortunately, people with this type of myopia tend to grow out of it as the eye develops with age.

Pathological Myopia

The rarest form of myopia and the cruelest. This type of myopia has two subcategories -- progressive and degenerative. Progressive myopia occurs when the eye is not only larger than normal, it also continues to grow. Degenerative myopia continues this trend; this name is given when progressive myopia begins to deteriorate the afflicted eyesight. These forms of myopia remain and progressively worsen as the victim ages.

General Causes of Myopia

Since myopia is not genetically inherited, you may wonder about other factors affecting myopia.

Poor posture is closely linked with myopia. Poor posture apparently causes the victim to carry tension in the body, which leads to strain and malfunction in eye development.

As mentioned previously, one line of thinking suggests that since children are forced to learn within the regimentation of the educational system, additional pressure and frustration can lead to eye strain that results in eye malformation. Thus, the way children study can influence the development of myopia.

Treating Myopia

Myopia is a condition that particularly highlights how lifestyle influences eyesight. The main cause of myopia is strain placed on the eyes. Hence, you have to learn how to not strain your eyes in order to stop these debilitating effects.

That said, you should practice looking further and further away (while taking appropriate breaks to relax) to see how much improvement you can make without pushing yourself to the point of further damage.

Those who suffer from myopia would do well to study this guide. The exercises found here will help train your eyes and offers significant help to those afflicted with this condition.

Presbyopia

As we grow older, age takes its toll on our organs. Many people find that after their fortieth birthday, they begin struggling to read that which they once were able to read before with ease. This is the after-effect of presbyopia -- the hardening of the lenses within the eyeball, resulting in partial reduction of vision.

Symptoms of Presbyopia
- Headache
- Difficulty seeing nearby objects and the manifestation of these symptoms when attempting to examine objects up close
- Fatigue
- Eye strain

Frequently, presbyopia is found with short-sightedness, far-sightedness or astigmatism. If you have any of these conditions you should beware of presbyopia.

Causes
As mentioned, presbyopia involves the hardening of the lenses. Since light contacts them incorrectly, images becomes blurred. Simply put, your eyes harden as you age, thus making it more difficult to focus on nearby objects.

Treatment of Presbyopia
There is no cure for presbyopia but there are ways to mitigate its effects. Most medical professionals will recommend the use of corrective aids -- typically bifocal glasses -- instead of considering natural alternatives to alleviate the suffering associated with presbyopia.

This guide has detailed exercises. Let me emphasize once again -- *take these exercises seriously*. They will help you adapt to the difficulty in focusing your eyesight. They also address damage done to the eye and even treat the changes in the eye caused by presbyopia.

Dyslexia

Who Does Dyslexia Impact?

Dyslexia can strike any one at any time. It affects adults and children and impacts lifestyle, whether it's you who has dyslexia or someone close to you. Many don't realize the strain of living with someone who has dyslexia can create constant pressure for everyone involved.

What is Dyslexia?

Have you ever read a number aloud only to realize you jumbled the digits? This can happen when you invert a phone number, or read 32 as 23. This can even occur with words, or "rdsow" to dyslexics. We all scramble the order of words or numbers sometimes but this occurs constantly with dyslexics.

Dyslexics suffer great mental anguish resulting from their condition, particularly since their problems with vision strains their eyes as they constantly attempt to keep the order of numbers and words straight.

Causes of Dyslexia

Dyslexia has multiple causes. Some people are born with this condition. In others it develops from undue pressure placed upon their reading comprehension as a child. Within the womb, if the fetus experiences brain damage the child will have a higher chance of being born dyslexic. These effects are similar at times to children born with mental developmental issues.

Children forced to continually read aloud (even when struggling to understand words or expressing frustration) have often been associated with strain and pressure linked to dyslexia. What started as misunderstood letters or numbers can easily become jumbled words or sentences.

Treatment for Dyslexia

The principal form of treatment for dyslexia is to remove learning pressure from the dyslexic individual. Easing pressure means not forcing them to read material that does not interest or frustrate them. The best way to alleviate this pressure is to simply relax -- even by using the techniques found in this guide.

Once relaxed, a dyslexic should use guide materials (like charts) that will help him/her identify individual letters and numbers without confusing their order.

Finally, give yourself time to work at this condition. It will not happen overnight and it will not be done if you rush or pressure yourself to be perfect. Make sure you are calm and relaxed. Then read at a pace that is comfortable for you. This strategy will offer you the best chance of overcoming dyslexia.

Floating Objects in Your Line of Vision

What are "floating objects in your line of vision"?

Floating specks are not a harmful condition. They may be associated with your eyes' ability to revive themselves, as some believe floating specks are dead cells you're disposing from your body. The term "floating specks" refers to those little 'objects' you sometimes see after you blink. They may come and go but you can get rid of them.

Do not forget: if they are a problem, seek medical attention. This guide is not a substitute for the guidance of a medical professional.

Causes of Floating Objects

As stated, current thinking indicates these objects are dead cells that the eye sheds. However, these episodes may last longer than just a few moments, thus becoming an extreme nuisance. Some factors that can lead to increased and prolonged floating objects are an unhealthy diet, alcohol abuse, stress or extreme fatigue.

Treating Floating Objects

Treat this condition by giving your eyes appropriate breaks and let yourself relax. As you repose, your eyes will naturally clear away dead cells. By using some of the exercises that focus on relaxing you will allow your eyes to naturally moisturize and rid itself of these floating objects.

Glaucoma

Glaucoma is unfortunately all too common yet remains largely unrecognized due to the lack of tests available for diagnosis. Optometrists can test for this affliction but since awareness is so low, many who suffer from glaucoma remain unaware of their condition.

What is Glaucoma?

Glaucoma feels like pressure on the eye, and is actually the process of the body slowly damaging the optic nerve to the point that it can no longer provide the eye with the nutrients it needs for regeneration.

What Are the Types of Glaucoma?

Like myopia, there are several different varieties of glaucoma. They are:

- Angle Closure Glaucoma (acute) – A form of glaucoma that appears very suddenly with symptoms of pain, blurry eyesight, nausea and redness. It occurs when the eye stops draining acqueous fluids.

  Acute glaucoma requires immediate medical attention, as it can cause permanent and irreversible damage if left untreated.

- Congenital Glaucoma – Congenital glaucoma, as the name implies, is present at or shortly after birth. Its symptoms include extremely watery eyes and sensitivity to light. Also, the eye has a cloudy appearance. This is one of the rarer forms and usually requires surgery.

- Open-Angle Glaucoma (chronic) – The most common of all of types.

- Secondary Glaucoma – This classification is a catch-all for damage that has occurred to the nerve as a result of other conditions or injuries. The sources of these injuries could be another condition (inflammation or cataracts, for example) or could even be something as simple as medication (steroids in particular).

Steroid use has been directly linked to the appearance of secondary glaucoma. It can place undue strain on the eye, resulting in severe damage.

Causes of Glaucoma

The fact that there are so many different varieties of glaucoma speaks volumes about the number of causes that can incur this condition. Some of the known agents include:

- Health conditions
- Inadequate drainage of aqueous fluid
- Insufficient blood flow
- Toxin build up
- Weak nerves around the eye

Treatment of Glaucoma

As with many eye maladies, glaucoma does not have a cure. However, there are treatments available. While these treatments vary, their aim is not to cure the issue but to rather manage the condition until there is nothing left to manage (i.e., the patient goes blind).

There are three primary levels of treatment – medical treatment, surgical intervention and alternative treatments. Each is addressed below.

Medical Treatments for Glaucoma

- Eye droplets – Medically prescribed eye drops can give some relief to those who suffer from glaucoma.
- Pills – Occasionally doctors will prescribe pills as an alternative to eye drops. These pills contain the same medication as eye drops.
- Puncturing of the eyeball – Eyeball puncturing is to be done **only by a medical professional** in order to ease the pressure that excess fluid can cause to those who suffer from glaucoma.

Surgical Intervention Methods

Surgery is typically prescribed when treatments are no longer slowing the progress of glaucoma and your physician fears further damage to the eye or potential vision loss. Treatment will be necessary in conjunction with surgery; these measures are merely means to maintain sight.

- Laser Trabeculoplasty
- Trabeculectomy Surgery – This surgery is the last resort (after laser trabeculoplasty). This surgery is an attempt to create a channel manually that allows proper drainage, alleviating pressure from undue buildup of acqueous liquid in the eye.

Alternative Glaucoma Treatments

- Relaxation techniques that work to improve circulation (see chapters on eye exercises for details).
- Close your eyes, tilt your head and expose yourself to light. Light, particularly when it conveys heat, can sometimes help clear blockages within the eye that may cause glaucoma-related issues.
- See dietary notes from previous chapters
- The palming exercise

Go Medical or Alternative?

Both the medical and alternative side of glaucoma treatment have valid options for treatment. As always, this guide recommends medical attention. We especially urge medical treatment because glaucoma is a condition that will likely require all options available, including both licensed physicians and natural measures.

If you are suffering from glaucoma, seek medical attention and advice BEFORE self-diagnosis or treatment!

Macular Degeneration

Vision naturally declines as people age and abuse their eyes. This happens because as we age, the blood vessels and arteries within the body harden and narrow, thus making it increasingly difficult for blood to reach required areas. Some people don't realize that blood carries nutrients. When areas of your body lack blood, they are starved of the nutrients that they need to run efficiently. This can lead to damage, and in the eyes this damage is called macular degeneration.

Who Does Macular Degeneration Affect?

Many people think that macular degeneration targets the elderly. However, macular degeneration begins when people are young – the effects are visible within the elderly. Put simply, the body has become damaged as a result of the macular degeneration present from a much earlier age.

What Is Macular Degeneration?

When the eyes decline to the point of damage -- specifically when the retina is damaged because of lack of nutrients -- this is called macular degeneration. It occurs when the eye is starved of the nutrient-laden blood it needs. The eye in particular needs nutrients to battle the buildup of toxins from within, as these toxins can kill parts of the eye. The lack of these nutrients causes toxins to accumulate and the eye thus becomes damaged.

Symptoms of Macular Degeneration
- Perceiving straight lines as curved
- Blurred vision
- Blindness (if left untreated)

Blurred vision is one of the first symptoms of macular degeneration, particularly when this blurriness appears near the center of the eye. However, if left untreated blurriness will be the least of the sufferer's problems, as blindness is a consequence of macular degeneration.

Causes of Macular Degeneration

Although macular degeneration is caused by the lack of blood flow to the eye, it is also caused by other influences related to lifestyle.

One of these influences is your level of physical activity. Sedentary lifestyles have been linked to macular degeneration. Sedentary lifestyle impacts the attitudes linked to this lifestyle and the diet that traditionally accompanies it.

Diet is the other leading cause of macular degeneration. A diet high in fats and oils can lead to arteriosclerosis that ultimately causes deficient blood flow -- the underlying problem.

You may have noticed how these factors are interconnected. A sedentary lifestyle is linked with poor diet, which is linked with arteriosclerosis, which is linked to blood deficiency, resulting in a buildup of toxins that cause macular degeneration. As the next section demonstrates, working with these factors will result in preventing macular degeneration rather than treating it.

Treating Macular Degeneration

There is no straightforward cure for macular degeneration, only prevention and treatment.

The best way to treat macular degeneration is to prevent it. This is accomplished by taking note of the risk factors that impact you and adjusting your lifestyle accordingly to help prevent damage.

However, as it may be too late at this point to prevent macular degeneration, let's discuss some treatment methods that may help in treating damage.

Diet

Avoid nicotine, foods high in caffeine, fried foods, fatty foods and dairy products. These foods have been linked to the clotting of arteries that starts the hardening process, causing difficulty for blood circulation.

Examples of these foods include milk, bacon, processed meats, doughnuts, fried foods, etc.

In contrast to avoidance strategies, you should eat foods that improve blood flow. Examples include good organic veggies, fruits and certain types of fish (salmon, tuna, sardines).

Other Ideas

There are other methods that help relieve macular degeneration. The following is a relatively comprehensive list.

- Attitude, attitude, attitude. Work on your attitude by fostering a positive outlook that raises your energy levels so you can follow the rest of these suggestions.
- Exercise on a regular basis – in particular cardio
- Relaxation
- Make use of the exercises in this guide that promote relaxation and increase blood flow to the eyes

By combining a good diet and these suggestions, you will help prevent further damage. Improving lifestyle is the key to battling macular degeneration.

As always, consult a doctor if suffering from macular degeneration.

Exercises to Improve Your Eyesight

All the conditions that we discussed can be addressed through effort, relaxation and exercise. We all treasure our eyesight, yet many people let it slip away without working to keep it. This guide presents several exercises to keep your eyesight at a healthy level and can even help regain vision loss caused by eye damage.

Before we begin, consider this suggestion: Work at your own pace! There is no pressure or rush. You risk eye strain by putting stress on yourself. It takes time to improve your vision -- it will come if you don't strain yourself. Don't be discouraged; you can do this if you put in the time it takes to do these simple exercises.

These exercises shouldn't be undertaken more than one at a time. Doing them singly will ensure that you understand what you're doing. You'll gain the benefits while measuring your progress.

<u>Exercise 1)</u> Improving Your Focus

Find someplace where you can see a fair distance away from you. This is where the exercise will take place. It can be outside, at the beginning of a long hallway or even from your window -- but remember you must be able to see a fairly long distance.

The Steps
Step 1) Find an object within three feet of where you are sitting/standing and focus on it. What is it? Examine it in detail. Once you've identified it, move on.

Step 2) Now pick something a little further away, but not too far -- perhaps about 25 - 30 feet distant. Focus on it as best you can. Notice as much detail as you can.

Step 3) Next, look in the distance (at least several hundred feet away) and focus on an object. A telephone pole, a rock or something you can't identify... yet. Now, do your best to figure out what it is.

Step 4) Find an object far away without moving closer to it. What is it? What do you notice about it?

This exercise is very easy and can be practiced in sets of ten, twice a day. It helps your ability to focus. An alternative version of this exercise is presented below.

Exercise 2) Improving Your Focus -- An Alternative

This version of the focus exercise can be done within the mind rather than space where you see far away and up close. It takes more imagination and indeed persistence but can be just as effective as the previous exercise.

The Steps

Step 1) Picture a shape. (Any shape -- circle, cube, cone, etc.) Imagine the shape is three feet away from you. Focus on it and once more, note what the object is and as much detail as you can see.

Step 2) Picture the shape moving away to a distance of 25 - 30 feet away. Again focus on it and think of all the details you can see.

Step 3) Again in your mind, place the shape several hundred feet away. How does it look now? Can you still notice what you could before? Remember, you cannot rely on the earlier memory of the object when it was closer to you. You must try to pretend this is an actual image in front of you.

Step 4) The final step involves moving the object even further away. How has your focus changed? How does it look when traveling away from you?

This exercise can also be done in sets of ten, twice a day, for best results.

Exercise 3) Improving Your Circulation

Efficient blood circulation is perhaps the most important thing you can do for your eyes. As previously mentioned, blood carries nutrients vital for organs throughout the body, protecting and preventing damage to the eyes.

The exercise below helps ensure that your circulation is effective and running smoothly.

The Steps
Step 1) Stand with your body completely relaxed, looking straight in front of you at all times.

Step 2) Look up at the ceiling, moving in a relaxed motion. Hold your gaze for a moment.

Step 3) Now shift your gaze to the floor, again, slowly moving your head at a relaxed pace.

Step 4) Repeat step 1.

This exercise should be done in sets of ten, twice a day.

<u>Exercise 4)</u> Improving Your Sight at a Distance

This exercise requires the use of a long, thin object (pen, finger, nail file, etc.). Ensure one of your eyes is closed at all times. This exercise works to help your eyesight adjust to different distances and seeing things in more detail, even when the objects are further away than you are accustomed to seeing.

The Steps

Step 1) Hold your chosen object up close to your face, about a palm's length away. Focus on the object, and only the object, for a few minutes.

Step 2) With the same eye open, shift your focus to an object some distance away. Focus on that for a moment.

Step 3) Return to step 1.

This exercise can be done in sets of twenty for each eye, throughout the day.

Exercise 5) Strengthening Your Eye Muscles

Strengthening your muscles improves your eyesight by increasing the flexibility of your gaze. Recall our discussion of presbyopia? Vision is reduced when the lens begins to harden but the reverse is true as well.

The Steps

Step 1) Picture a large figure 8. Place it in your mind approximately ten feet away from your body, paying particular notice to its size.

Step 2) Slowly watch as the figure turns on its side towards you.

Step 3) Slowly trace the figure 8's complete form clockwise, appreciating each curve and moving at a relaxed pace. (This can be very relaxing.)

Step 4) Now start to trace backwards (counter-clockwise), again moving slowly and in a relaxed motion.

Step 5) Rest your eyes and allow time to relax.

This exercise should be done in sets of four, twice a day.

Exercise 6) Using Your Hands to Help Relax Your Eyes

This exercise is one of the most relaxing exercises to do because you are actually giving your eyes time to relax (if done correctly). The more accustomed you become to taking time from your day to relax the better you will be at this exercise – and the more you will appreciate it.

This exercise can be particularly useful for people who have no more than just a moment in their busy day to break away from their activities and give their eyes a much needed break. You will love how refreshed you feel after you master this task!

The Steps

Step 1) Remove any corrective aids (glasses, contacts, etc.) and take a few deep breaths. Make sure you are in a comfortable position.

Step 2) Lean towards your knees (or a desk if you're seated at one) and use your elbows to support yourself.

Step 3) Begin rubbing the palms of your hands together until they feel pleasantly warm.

Step 4) Take your now-warmed hands and gently cup your eyes. Be sure to avoid placing undue pressure or stress on your eyes. This will create a cover that allows your eyes to still move, but gives them a break from the stimulation surrounding you.

Step 5) Slowly tense and then relax your muscles throughout your body. Feel the effect it has on your eyes, and the deep level of darkness that now covers your lids.

Note: The less light you see, the more relaxed you are!

Stay in this position for 10-15 minutes.

Step 6) Slowly open your eyes. Recognize how this rejuvenation makes a difference to your vision. You likely see clearer, and no doubt feel much more relaxed.

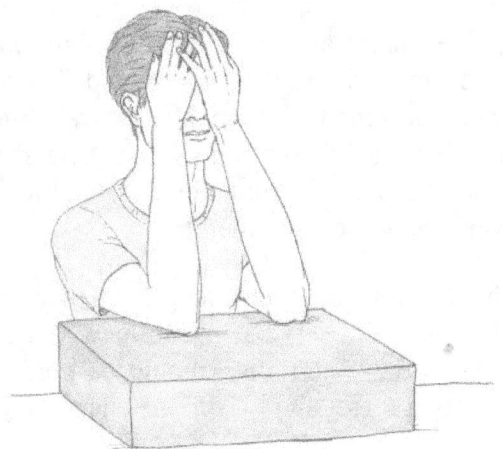

A Picture Demonstrating the Exercise

This exercise should be done whenever you have time available. Be certain that if this exercise was for relaxation alone it would be worth the effort. The fact that it improves your eyesight and protects vision is an absolute bonus. These benefits should encourage you to do this exercise as often as possible.

Exercise Using Charts

The following five charts are from Dr. William Bates, a famous ophthalmologist from New York who created The Bates Method. These charts were designed to help people train their eyes more efficiently by combining the body's need for exercise and relaxation to improve vision. They are not intended to frustrate or discourage anyone -- and yes, you too can do them!

These charts should be printed and hung someplace where you can readily see them. They will serve as a reminder to keep a routine in using them. Each of these activities should be performed regularly and always from several feet away from the chart.

In the beginning you may feel as though your eyesight is terrible. But you're already working to improve your vision just by reading this book! Follow the tips, do the exercises and (critically) track your progress so you can measure the difference your diligence makes in improving your eyesight!

Over time your vision will work better and you will even be able to compete with yourself by doing these exercises.

For each of the charts, follow the series of steps provided and you will be well on your way to improving your vision. Take notes so you can track your progress!

Chart Instructions
Step 1) Make sure the space surrounding the charts is satisfactory. The area should be well lit and someplace you frequently access. This will encourage you to practice your exercises.

Step 2) Moving from the top down, read as many individual letters as you can.

Step 3) Use the palm of your hand to cover one eye and try to read the charts again, seeing how far you can get until you can no longer progress.

Step 4) Repeat step three using the other eye.

To get printable versions of the eye exercise charts, please visit: www.improvevisionnaturally.com/join/

Bonus Exercise – Pinhole Glasses

Light impacts our eyes. The right amount allows you to see but too much light can cause blurred vision since excess light dilates your pupil (as a way of protecting your eyes). There are ways to correct the blurred aspect of your vision; one of the best methods is the use of pinhole glasses.

The best part of using these glasses? No optometrist's prescription is necessary! Simple to make, you can use them during those opportune moments when full vision is not required.

Creating Your Own Pinhole Glasses
Materials:
- Card stock
- Old glasses
- Pins
- Tape
- Screwdriver

Directions:
1) With the aid of a screwdriver, remove the lenses from an old pair of glasses you saved for just this purpose.
2) Use the lenses as stencils on the card stock. Use the old lenses as a template to ensure the new lenses fit the frames of the glasses.
3) Poke between 66 - 76 pinholes into the stencils, keeping the holes spaced as evenly as possible.
4) Cut the stencils carefully. Remember they have to fit into the old frames. Be prepared to make modifications if necessary.
5) Tape the new lenses to the old frames
6) See that the lenses fit and the tape does not cover any pinholes.

It is worth noting that the effects will seem odd to you the first few times you wear these glasses. We are accustomed to seeing the world in large sweeping glances. When your vision is restricted you may become disoriented. Don't force yourself to wear the glasses for too long so you won't strain your vision.

Why Wear Pinhole Glasses?

Pinhole glasses help darken your eyes except for the tiny pinholes of focused light. This lack of light dilates the pupils yet still protects the eyes from damage while allowing you to benefit from your now-focused attention. Your vision seems much sharper when you only focus on what is directly before you. This is a simple vision exercise that can help improve your eyesight dramatically.

*Caution: Do **NOT** wear these while engaged in any activity that requires full vision – this means '**NO DRIVING**'!*

Improving Your Eyesight with Diet

While we've spent much time discussing eye improvement exercises, we would be remiss if we did not consider the impact of diet. Diet is an example of a lifestyle factor that is worth changing for the sake of your vision and is certainly worth the investment of time. People don't usually associate diet with vision but it's a fact that a poor diet deprives the body of nutrients just as sure as hardening of arteries does.

How can improving your diet help enhance your eyesight? The short answer -- by time and effort. Your diet is a habit built over years and its effects will not be reversed overnight. But by making the effort to do your exercises and taking these tips seriously you can reverse some of this damage.

This does not mean you're doomed to a starvation-based diet. This guide lists foods that help improve eyesight naturally. The biggest caveat is to vary these edibles from time to time so your body receives the maximum nutrients available.

Foods You Should Avoid

Before mentioning foods recommended for good eyesight, let us caution you about some foods and habits to avoid. The list below contains items bad for your health, not just vision. You will notice an improvement in both your health and eyesight if you eliminate them from your diet.

- Alcohol
- Bakery products (pastries, cookies, doughnuts)
- Fried foods (fast food, fried chicken, anything cooked in grease)
- Nicotine (cigars, tobacco, cigarettes)
- Oils

- Processed meats (bacon, ham, pepperoni)
- Red meat (beef, pork)

After seeing some of your favorite foods you may be inclined to dismiss this lifestyle change. Don't make this mistake! While totally eliminating these items from your body is the healthiest option, you can receive considerable benefits just by reducing your intake of them.

Make a doughnut a treat instead of a habitual morning pick-me-up. Indulge in alcohol only on occasion. Try some of these tips and see how your body reacts. We should point out that the elimination of these items requires you to replace these poor foods with healthier choices. The next section looks at foods that are good for your eyesight and health.

Foods That Are Good for You

Fish -- Great for Your Eyesight (and Your Diet!)

- Fish high in omega fatty acids are particularly helpful for your diet
- Albacore Tuna
- Mackerel
- Salmon
- Sardines

Spices to Add to Your Diet

- Dill
- Oregano
- Parsley
- Turmeric

Fruits That Are Good For Your Eyesight

- Acerola
- Bilberries

- Blueberries
- Cantaloupe
- Dried Apricots
- Guavas
- Kiwi
- Lemons

Veggies That Are Good For Your Eyesight

- Broccoli
- Brussel sprouts
- Carrots
- Celery
- Chili
- Collard Greens
- Corn
- Green beans
- Kale
- Leek
- Lettuce
- Mustard Greens
- Peas
- Spinach
- Squash
- Sweet potatoes
- Tomatoes
- Yams

Now that you know great food is available that is also good for you, you may be more willing to make the dietary alterations to help your eyesight. It is worth noting that reducing unhealthy foods will not just help your vision but also your health. However, we understand diet is a personal lifestyle choice.

The bottom line: keep your junk food intake to a minimum and your healthy food intake varied and frequent. When you combine the power of diet and exercise you will be well on your way to improving your vision.

Check out www.CompleteVisionHealth.com, for total eye care essential nutrition.

Herbs and Herbal Remedies

Herbs can be a great aid in healing the body and improving eyesight. Herbal remedies have become exceedingly popular in recent years; this chapter overviews some popular herbs available to you that combats the damage of eye strain.

Again, this is not a substitute for medical advice. Seek the advice of a medical practitioner (or even an herbalist); do not JUST rely on this book.

Aspalathus

The effects of Aspalathus are similar to those of Bilberry.
This South African herb, also known as Rooibos, is high in antioxidants. Antioxidants are well known for their ability to promote the health of eyesight as well as the immune system because of their blood cleansing properties.

Bilberry

In addition to its high levels of antioxidants, Bilberry also contains a specific ingredient which is the root of its herbal powers -- anthocyanosides (a type of bioflavonoids). This ingredient is important because it has been directly linked to improvement in those with macular degeneration, a condition discussed earlier in this book.

In addition to the conditions Bilberry treats, it has also been known to increase its user's clarity and range of eyesight. In other words, you will be able to see faraway distances again.

Warning: Bilberry effects are far-reaching but insufficient to reverse far-sightedness, short-sightedness or cataracts unless combined with other approaches to vision improvement.

Bilwa

Bilwa has been linked with the treatment of conjunctivitis and sties in particular. If you suffer from these conditions we strongly recommend you add this to your diet.

Ginkgo Biloba

Gingko biloba (like bilberry) is used to treat macular degeneration.

Like passionflower, ginkgo biloba helps clear the circulatory system so that more blood can reach required parts of the body. It actually works to counteract existing damage, making it especially useful for those who suffer from conditions resulting from circulatory problems.

Golden Seal

Golden seal is primarily a painkiller for your eyes. It helps to reduce pain, irritation and inflammation in the eye. Being a natural substance, golden seal is a safer option than many other remedies.

Mahonia Grape Extract

This herb is superb protecting the eye from future damage. Its elements work together to strengthen the eye and protect it from sunlight exposure and damage that normally results from the aging process.

Passionflower

This herb has been linked to efficient blood flow throughout the body. It helps to dilate the blood vessels, which allows the passage of more blood and thus more nutrients. This can be a tremendous help in relieving the daily strain we put on our eyes.

In Conclusion

The herbs listed above have two common elements: they all are linked to some specific benefit for your eyesight and they are all herbs and thus a natural alternative to medications or other methods of helping your eyesight. Herbs have the added benefit of a long history of treatment as part of the healing process.

If herbal remedies interest you, do some research or contact an herbalist for more information.

Keep in mind that using herbs is only a part of the strategy involved in maintaining good eyesight. Herbs are but a single component of diet. They need to be combined with eye exercises and relaxation to be effective in protecting your sight.

Check out www.CompleteVisionHealth.com, for total eye care essential nutrition.

Using Juices to Help Restore Your Sight

This book has outlined a number of conditions and sources of damage to the eye as well as several exercises that can help treat debilitating vision problems. But did you know juice can also help? Not sugary junk food type juices but a fruit or vegetable juice (which can be just as refreshing).

Many people have bought into the juicing craze, excited about this delicious tasting vitamin delivery system, but even these converts may not always realize the benefits to their vision when drinking these types of juice.

This chapter outlines different types of juice and how each can be used to combat the effects of various vision maladies. Before mentioning different types of juice , let's first look at exactly why you should drink fruit and vegetable juice.

Why Juice Is So Great

Juice is easily absorbed by the body. This means that you can reap the benefits of juice easier than eating certain foods containing the same nutrients!

Drinking fruit/veggie juice also helps your digestive system by providing needed digestive enzymes. These enzymes are responsible for breaking down foods. The more you have, the more efficiently your body can break down food and continue the digestive process.

Bottoms up! The following sections reviews juicer recipes known for helping with certain eye conditions.

Best's Disease

This recipe should be mainly comprised of vegetables.

- Apples
- Beets
- Cabbage
- Carrots
- Chlorophyll
- Celery
- Garlic
- Ginger
- Grapes
- Leek
- Lemon
- Parsley
- Raspberries
- Spinach
- Wheat grass

Cataracts (and Conjunctivitis)

- Apple
- Blueberry
- Carrot
- Celery
- Endive
- Parsley
- Spinach

Diabetic Retinopathy

- Asparagus
- Beets
- Cabbage
- Carrots
- Celery
- Chlorophyll
- Garlic
- Ginger
- Jerusalem artichokes
- Leek

- Parsley
- Pumpkin
- Spinach

Floating Objects in Your Line of Vision
This recipe should be comprised of mostly vegetables.

- Apple
- Beets
- Carrots
- Celery
- Garlic
- Parsley
- Parsnip
- Raspberries

Glaucoma

- Apple
- Beets
- Cabbage
- Carrots
- Celery
- Cucumber
- Parsley
- Plums
- Radish
- Turnip

Leber's Optic Nerve Atrophy, Optic Neuritis

- Beets
- Berries

- Cabbage
- Carrots
- Chlorophyll
- Endive
- Ginger
- Parsley
- Wheat grass

Macular Degeneration

- Apples
- Bell peppers (green and red)
- Broccoli
- Greens
- Raspberries

Retinitis Pigmentosis

This recipe should be comprised of mostly veggies

- Beets
- Cabbage
- Chlorophyll
- Garlic
- Ginger
- Grapes
- Leek
- Lemon
- Parsley
- Raspberries
- Spinach
- Wheat grass

How to Make the Most Out of Juice

Mix and match and find what tastes good. The best way to get the most out of juice is to drink it regularly! The following tips will help you maximize nutritional value from your juice.

- Use fresh fruits and vegetables and go organic where possible. Organic fruits and vegetables are significantly better for the body than fruits and vegetables sprayed with pesticides. While pesticides are effective in repelling pests, these toxins can be harmful to the body.
- Filter out the fiber in your juice. Filtering makes juice even easier to digest, and many pesticides bond to fiber. Removing fiber makes your juice even better for you.
- Make sure to drink your greens – literally. Foods like broccoli, kale, spinach and other quality green vegetables should comprise most of your juice.
- Try adding whole grains (yeast, wheat germ, etc.) to your juice to ensure you are not only getting the nutrients of the juice but also the protein that comes with a meal. This is a great way to get the full benefit of juice.
- Check the speed of your juicer. Juicers come in a variety of speeds but some of the most common range from 80 rpm up to 3600 rpm. We recommend purchasing a juicer that functions at no higher than 80 rpm because at this speed the juicer can do its job but will not damage or destroy any nutrients in the fruits and vegetables. This may not be the advice you receive from the retailer (where ease of cleaning and short processing times rule) but it is better for you in the long run.
- Make as much juice as you need... right now. The enzymes that benefit your digestive tract in juice do not necessarily age well and some break down when exposed to light. This means the best way to get maximum advantage from your juice is to immediately drink what you make!

Summary of Tips

We've provided many natural treatments for you to improve your vision. Since we encourage you to review as necessary to make sure you understand each exercise, let's summarize how you can improve your vision.

Here's to healthy vision!

Air Conditioners – Air conditioners are fine to use for your comfort but when they are aimed straight at your face, your eyes will dry out quickly. This can lead to discomfort, dryness and can increase your vulnerability to scratches on the eye.

Dietary Considerations – When you eat junk you're not just ingesting unhealthy substances, you're preventing your body from getting the vitamins and minerals it needs to function. So our tip for improving your vision with regards to diet? Eat well! This will help your body, mind and sight!

Eye Breaks – We have shown several exercises involving breaks from prolonged exposure to computer screens, concentration and stress. Taking time out can help reverse the damage you've already done.

Exercises – Exercise is great for the body so why wouldn't it be great for your sight? We've provided many exercises throughout this guide to help you to keep your eyes moisturized and strong.

Quit Smoking – Smoking is unhealthy for you in many ways. From burning your lungs and ingesting toxins to cataracts and other forms of vision damage, it is absolutely in your best interest to quit smoking immediately. It may seem fun but it is definitely not worth it.

Salt – Remember this about salt: too much of a good thing CAN hurt! Try substituting salt with a variety of spices that add flavor to your food. You'll protect your vision without damaging your health.

Sunglasses – Sunglasses can be a great way to protect your eyes from the sun's harmful rays. Well-made sunglasses are coated with extra protection to safeguard your eyes and keep them from the ultraviolet rays of the sun. This is a preventative rather than an improvement method.

The Best Tip? Heed the Advice in This Book! These tips have been compiled to help you to improve your health and vision. Read this book and personalize the tips for your own lifestyle. By making optimal use of these tips you will reverse existing damage and prevent future harm.

You will be stunned to find how working to improve your vision actually works to improve your life.

Conclusions

I hope you've enjoyed this guide. You are now armed with knowledge that can help you improve your vision naturally. Feel free to re-read relevant chapters or summarize the exercises and post them somewhere as a reminder to do them. Ideally you should work to help relax your eyes every single day!

Remember that improving vision is a lifestyle move; it may take some effort to reverse the damage you've done. Similarly, because it's a lifestyle move, performing these exercises do not create instant miracles.

Understanding the facts above will help you establish realistic expectations of progress and empower you to move forward. There is nothing in your life (not age, gender or the time spent in using corrective aids) that disqualifies you from improving your eyesight.

You can improve your vision if you want!

Now that you have a blueprint, it's up to you to make the improvements. If you do, I am confident that not only will your vision improve, but so will your overall health and well-being. You will SEE the difference.

Please remember this guide does not substitute for advice from a physician or optometrist.

Thank you for reading "How To Improve Your Vision Naturally: Strategies and Exercises to Restore Your Eyesight"

Resources

To get other exclusive bonuses and special offers, please visit the following website:

www.SparrowPublication.com